What you really need to know about

BREAST
CANCER

Dr. Robert Buckman

with Dr. Tereza Whittaker

Introduced by John Cleese

LEBHAR-FRIEDMAN BOOKS

New York • Chicago • Los Angeles • London • Paris • Tokyo

Lebhar-Friedman Books
425 Park Avenue
New York, NY 10022

A Marshall Edition
Conceived by Marshall Editions
The Orangery
161 New Bond Street
London W1Y 9PA

First U.S. edition published 2000 by Lebhar-Friedman Books.

First published in the UK in 2000 by Marshall Publishing Ltd.
Copyright © 2000 Marshall Editions Developments Ltd.

Library of Congress Cataloging-in-Publication Data
on file at the Library of Congress

ISBN 0-86730-826-5

Originated in Italy by Articolor
Printed in and bound in Italy by Milanostampa

Project Editor Alison Murdoch
Additional Editing Jill Cropper
U.S. Editor Maggi McCormick
Indexer Stephen Fall
Art Editor Louise Morley
Illustrator Coral Mula
Picture Research Vickie Walters
Managing Editor Anne Yelland
Managing Art Editor Helen Spencer
Editorial Director Ellen Dupont
Art Director Dave Goodman
Editorial Coordinator Ros Highstead
D.T.P. Editor Lesley Gilbert
Production Nikki Ingram, Anna Pauletti

Cover photography: front GJ Images/The Image Bank; back GJ Images/The Image Bank

The consultant for this book was Shari Leipzig, M.D., who is an obstetrician and gynecologist in general practice
in New York City. She is also a clinical instructor of obstetrics and gynecology at Mt. Sinai School of Medicine.

Contents

Foreword

Most of you know me best as someone who makes people laugh.

But for 30 years I've also been involved with communicating information. And one particular area in which communication often breaks down is the doctor/patient relationship. We have all come across doctors who fail to communicate clearly, using complex medical terms when a simple explanation would do, and dismiss us with a "come back in a month if you still feel unwell." Fortunately I met Dr Robert Buckman.

Rob is one of North America's leading experts on cancer, but far more importantly he is a doctor who believes that hiding behind medical jargon is unhelpful and unprofessional. He wants his patients to understand what is wrong with them, and spends many hours with them—and their families and close friends—making sure they understand everything. Together we created a series of videos, with the jargon-free title *Videos for Patients*. Their success has prompted us to write books that explore medical conditions in the same clear, simple terms.

This book is one of a series that will tell you all you need to know about your condition. It assumes nothing. If you have a helpful, honest, communicative doctor, you will find here the extra information that he or she simply may not have time to tell you. If you are less fortunate, this book will help to give you a much clearer picture of your situation.

More importantly—and this was a major factor in the success of the videos—you can access the information here again and again. Turn back, read over, until you really know what your doctor's diagnosis means. In addition, because in the middle of a consultation you may not think of everything you would like to ask your doctor, you can also use the book to help you formulate the questions you would like to discuss with him or her.

John Cleese

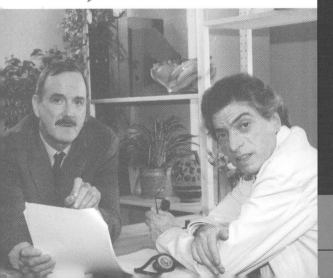

Introduction

Breast cancer is the most common form of cancer in women, affecting one in eight North American women during their lifetimes. The likelihood of developing it becomes greater as you get older, and it is most likely of all to develop in women who are past menopause.

Information and support

As with most cancers, the earlier breast cancer is detected and diagnosed, the better the chances are of successful treatment. One of the best ways of making sure that breast cancer is spotted as early as possible is to check your breasts once a month. By doing this, you become familiar with their usual appearance, contour, and feel, and are thus better able to seek early medical advice if there are any changes in either breast that are out of the ordinary. This book also gives you information about other symptoms and signs that could indicate breast cancer prompting you to see your doctor at an early stage in the disease.

The most serious problem with breast cancer is that it may spread to distant parts of the body. Doctors are not able to predict precisely whether a particular breast cancer will spread, but there are certain features that indicate whether the chance of spreading is high or low. On the pages that follow, you can read about the different types of breast cancer, how doctors estimate the chance of spread, and the various treatments you may be offered.

Exploring treatment options

For most women, the first treatment is surgery to remove the lump in their breast. The treatment given after this very much depends on the chance of the cancer spreading. You may be offered radiation therapy, chemotherapy, or hormone therapy, or a combination of treatments. This book tells you why each treatment may be offered, its beneficial effects, and also the possible side effects you may experience. Armed with this knowledge, you can make an informed choice about your treatment—if you know that your cancer has a high chance of spreading and a particular treatment can reduce that chance, you may be more likely to accept it if your doctor recommends it. If the chance of spread is low, and therefore the chance that you have already been cured by surgery is high, you may be less motivated to accept more treatment. It is always your choice.

A normal life

Remaining as healthy as you can will be one of your prime concerns after breast cancer. You will be given exercises to help you regain mobility in your arm and shoulder after surgery, and you should not be afraid to ask for any help you may need to deal with the anxiety and depression that can occur after cancer treatment. Looking good is important, too. An attractive wig and a good prosthesis—if you need them—can do wonders for your self-esteem and help you get on with this new phase of your life.

Y-ME BREAST CANCER CENTER

This organization offers information and support to all those affected by breast cancer or who have breast health concerns. It runs a telephone helpline and has a Web site full of practical advice and news on the latest research. Details can be found on page 78.

Chapter

1

SYMPTOMS & CAUSES

What is breast cancer?

A cancer is a group of abnormal cells growing together in an uncontrolled way, invading and damaging healthy tissue. A group of growing cancer cells forms a lump, which is called a tumor. If the tumor is in the breast, it is called breast cancer.

Cells are the body's building blocks—all of our organs and tissues are made up of many different types of cells. The body keeps itself healthy through cell growth and renewal, and almost all cells need to be replaced at regular intervals. Normal, healthy cells grow, divide, and die under the control of genes. If there is a change (mutation) in any of the growth-controlling genes, a healthy cell turns into an unhealthy tumor cell. These changes make the cell look abnormal when it is seen under a microscope. In addition to changing shape, the cells behave differently. They grow uncontrollably and divide to form more and more tumor cells.

Tumors can be benign or malignant. Benign tumors grow slowly, do not spread to other parts of the body, and are not life-threatening. Malignant tumors are harmful. They grow more rapidly, and the cells may spread to other parts of the body where they form secondary tumors (also known as metastatic tumors).

The structure of the breast

The breasts are made up of glandular tissue held together by connective tissue and fat. The glandular tissue consists of lobules and ducts. During breast feeding, the lobules fill with milk that then flows along the ducts leading to the nipple. The ducts and lobules are supported by the connective tissue. Breasts change through a woman's life. Young women have more glandular tissue than older women, making their breasts firmer. As women get older, the proportion of fat in their breasts increases, and the breasts tend to droop more.

The breasts sit on top of the chest muscles, outside the rib cage. The arteries carry oxygen-rich blood to the breasts, while the veins drain the blood away. This draining of blood through the veins sometimes provides a route for breast cancer to spread through the body.

The lymphatic system

The breast also has a lymphatic system, which plays an important role in filtering harmful substances. It consists of lymph nodes (the main ones are in the neck, armpits, and groin) linked by vessels that contain a fluid called lymph. Lymph flows around the body in these vessels in the same way that blood flows in the veins and arteries.

YOU REALLY NEED TO KNOW

◆ The body is made up of cells. Normal, healthy cells can turn into abnormal cells, and a group of abnormal cells is called a cancer.

◆ Tumor is another word for a lump, which can be benign or malignant.

◆ Benign tumors grow slowly and do not spread through the body.

◆ Malignant tumors are more serious than benign tumors but in many cases, they can be treated successfully.

UNDER THE SKIN

Chest wall

Fat

The breast consists of glandular lobules and ducts held together by connective tissue and fat.

Connective tissue

Duct

Nipple

Lobule

What is breast cancer?

What is breast cancer?

Screening refers to tests done to look for cancer. These include breast examination and special X-rays called mammograms.

Remission is when cancer has responded to treatment and is under control. It is not the same as being cured, but if a cancer stays away for more than 10 years, it may be considered cured.

Women and cancer

One in three people in the world will develop some form of cancer during their lifetime, and in women, this cancer is most likely to be cancer of the breast. Thirty percent of cancers (one in three) diagnosed in women are breast cancer. Lung cancer, cancer of the colon or large intestine, uterine cancer, and leukemia are the next most common cancers affecting women.

Is breast cancer on the increase?

In North America, approximately one in eight women of all ages will develop breast cancer at some time in her life, and about 195,000 new cases are diagnosed each year. Many people are worried that breast cancer is becoming more widespread, because a few years ago the figure quoted was one in twelve women. The disease

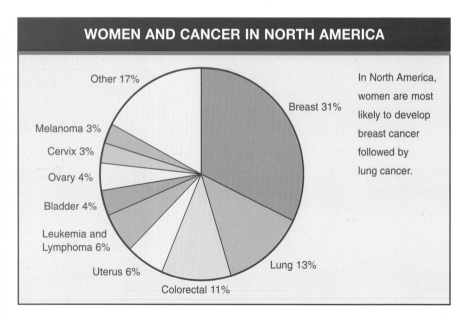

WOMEN AND CANCER IN NORTH AMERICA

Other 17%
Melanoma 3%
Cervix 3%
Ovary 4%
Bladder 4%
Leukemia and Lymphoma 6%
Uterus 6%
Colorectal 11%
Lung 13%
Breast 31%

In North America, women are most likely to develop breast cancer followed by lung cancer.

is, in fact, becoming a little more common, but some of this increase may be explained by the success of screening programs in diagnosing breast cancer at a much earlier stage than was previously possible. It is not entirely clear why the rate of breast cancer is so high in the Western world, but we do know that the Western lifestyle plays a role (see p. 14).

Who gets breast cancer?

The overwhelming majority of breast cancers occur in women—more than 99 percent. The next most important risk factor is a woman's age. The disease is found more frequently in older women. At the age of 25, the risk of developing breast cancer is approximately one in 20,000. By 35, this number increases to one in about 600, and at age 50 the risk is one in 50.

Older women who have passed menopause are the most likely of all to get breast cancer. This is why breast cancer screening programs are aimed at older women. The American College of Radiology recommends an annual mammogram beginning at age 40. (In Canada, mammography is advised every two years from age 50.) Screening mammograms aim to pick up cancer as early as possible, before the tumor has had time to grow and spread. The sooner a tumor is found and cancer diagnosed, the better the chances of treating it successfully.

What is the outlook?

Although breast cancer can be a life-threatening disease, if it is detected early enough, when the cancer is still small and before it has had a chance to spread to other parts of the body, up to 80 percent of women will be treated successfully and cured.

YOU REALLY NEED TO KNOW

◆ Breast cancer is the most common form of cancer to affect women.

◆ The risk of developing breast cancer increases with age, and it is most common in post-menopausal women.

◆ If breast cancer is detected early, there is a good chance that it can be cured.

What is breast cancer?

Causes of breast cancer

✓ Nearly two-thirds of women with breast cancer have no identifiable risk factors for developing the disease. Ninety percent of women who develop breast cancer have no family history of the disease.

✓ There is no evidence that low-energy radiation, such as that from a computer screen, increases a woman's risk of developing breast cancer. The X-rays used in mammography are also safe.

No one knows for sure what causes breast cancer. We do know that the disease is much more common in countries where people have a Western lifestyle than it is in developing countries. However, we do not know precisely what it is about the lifestyle in these countries that causes women to develop breast cancer. There is some evidence to suggest that it is partly due to diet—particularly the higher proportion of fat in the food we eat—but more research needs to be done.

Even though we do not know exactly how breast cancer is caused, we do know some of the things—the risk factors—that make a particular woman more liable than the average woman in her country to develop breast cancer. Being exposed to a risk increases your chances of developing cancer, but not everyone in a high-risk group will automatically do so.

Increasing age

Age alone does not cause cancer, but the incidence of breast cancer increases the older you get. Eighty percent of breast cancers occur in women over 50. It may be that initial damage to cells took place many years previously, and that the cancer took time to develop.

Age at first pregnancy

If you have your first child when you are young—before the age of about 18—you have a lower chance of developing breast cancer. We do not know why this is, and it does not necessarily mean that early pregnancy is a good idea. Having a child at such a young age can have serious consequences of its own. And, the protection against breast cancer is only partial—it is a weak protector rather than a total preventer.

INCIDENCE OF BREAST CANCER

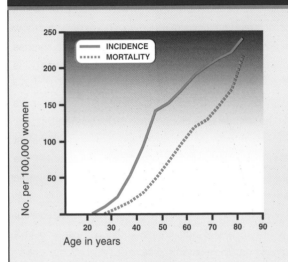

INCIDENCE
MORTALITY

No. per 100,000 women

250
200
150
100
50

20 30 40 50 60 70 80 90

Age in years

Age is the most important risk factor for developing breast cancer, and incidence increases dramatically with age.

Number of menstrual cycles

The total number of menstrual cycles you have in your life is related to your risk of getting breast cancer, because it affects your exposure to the hormone estrogen. If your periods start when you are young and your menopause occurs late, the overall number of years of exposure to estrogen is higher than for women who have a later first period and earlier menopause. This is known to increase the risk of developing breast cancer. In China, for example, where breast cancer is rare, the average age of the onset of periods is 17 years; in much of the Western world, including North America, it is 12 years.

YOU REALLY NEED TO KNOW

◆ No one knows for sure what causes breast cancer.

◆ A number of risk factors are known to increase your chance of developing breast cancer, but they don't inevitably lead to your developing the condition. Some of these factors are beyond your control.

Causes of breast cancer

Causes of breast cancer

Estrogen and progesterone are the two main female hormones. Estrogen influences cell division in the breast, and it is this effect that is thought to be important in the development of breast cancer.

Smoking is linked with other cancers, such as cervical cancer, and there are studies suggesting that it plays a role in breast cancer.

Breastfeeding

Women of all ages who breastfeed their babies gain a small amount of protection against breast cancer. But some research suggests that even this is not noticeable unless breastfeeding has continued for several years—far longer than most women in the West breastfeed.

A previous breast lump

Lumps in the breast are very common. Most non-cancerous lumps in younger women are caused by benign tumors called fibroadenomas. In older women, noncancerous breast lumps are more likely to be caused by cysts.

Neither fibroadenomas nor cysts normally pose any health risks and do not increase the chance of getting cancer later. However, if a benign breast lump shows certain changes, called atypical hyperplasia (see p. 19), when looked at under a microscope, there seems to be a slight increase in the chance that the woman will later develop breast cancer, even though that particular lump has been removed. Experts believe that atypical hyperplasia is a sign that the cells in the breast are generally unstable, so there is a greater-than-average chance that later on another part of the breast (or part of the other breast) will develop a cancer.

Can the pill cause breast cancer?

The available evidence suggests that the contraceptive pill probably does not contribute to the development of breast cancer, and certainly not if you take it for less than 10 years. What matters is the dose of estrogen in the pill, and modern pills contain much lower doses than earlier pills. Although there may be a small increase in risk with long-term use, the benefits of the pill, which include protection against ovarian cancer, still definitely outweigh the risks.

Prolonged use of any estrogen therapy, including hormone replacement therapy (HRT), taken to protect against the effects of menopause, may increase the risk of breast cancer very slightly. In the past, HRT contained high doses of estrogen, but modern versions use much smaller doses, and there does not seem to be any increased risk of breast cancer in the first 10 years of use. Estrogen also protects against heart disease and osteoporosis, which may pose a much greater threat to life and health than any increased risk of breast cancer.

RUNNING IN THE FAMILY

◆ A woman with a first-degree relative (mother or sister) who had breast cancer is twice as likely to develop the disease compared with someone with no family history of breast cancer. If that relative suffered from breast cancer at a young age, i.e. before menopause, the relative risk is greater. Women whose aunts or grandmothers had breast cancer also have an increased risk, but to a lesser extent.

◆ Two genes, labeled BRCA1 and BRCA2, which are probably present in fewer than one in 20 women, indicate that a woman has about an 80-percent chance of developing breast cancer and a 50-percent chance of passing the gene on to her daughters. Gene testing is not routinely available, but it might be worthwhile to test women in families with a high incidence of breast cancer to check for either of these genes.

YOU REALLY NEED TO KNOW

◆ Taking a contraceptive pill for less than 10 years does not increase the risk of developing breast cancer.

◆ Using HRT or another form of estrogen therapy might increase the risk of developing breast cancer, but estrogen therapy does offer protection against heart disease and osteoporosis.

Causes of breast cancer

Types of breast cancer

Cancer of the breast can be classified in many different ways, depending on what the cells look like under a microscope. Not all of the visible differences affect the way the cancer behaves and so do not influence the choice of treatment, but one feature is of great importance—whether the cancer is invasive or not.

Invasive disease

Breast cancer begins inside either one of the ducts of the breast or one of the lobules. With invasive cancer, the pathologist (who studies the cells under the microscope) can see the cancer going through the wall of the duct or through the lobule out into the surrounding breast tissue. "Invasive breast cancer" means cancer that is spreading out of the duct or out of the lobule in which it first developed. Most breast cancers are of the invasive type.

Non-invasive disease

Some cancers stay inside the ducts or lobules. These are called "in situ" (Latin for "in the original position"). In-situ cancers behave differently from the more common invasive cancers and may not cause any further trouble once they have been removed. They are also treated differently from the invasive types of breast cancer.

Ductal carcinoma in situ (DCIS) can grow as a small lump in just one place, or it can develop in more than one duct or part of a duct. Lobular carcinoma in situ (LCIS) is cancer growing inside one of the lobules. Although an in-situ cancer tends not to become invasive itself, if a woman does develop one, it means there is an increased risk of her developing another cancer elsewhere in the breast in the future.

Premalignant disease

Normal cells grow, divide, and die in a regular way. Sometimes an overgrowth of normal-looking cells form a lump called hyperplasia. Although this condition is harmless, it can lead to atypical hyperplasia, where the cells lose their normal shape and appearance. Atypical hyperplasia is also usually benign, but some types may be premalignant—a warning sign that cancer may develop.

Other types of breast cancer

Other, rarer types of breast cancer include Paget's disease, where a slow-growing cancer produces changes in the nipple; cystic carcinoma, which is a cancer growing within a cyst; and inflammatory cancer of the breast, which causes redness, swelling, and pain. It spreads quickly, and often there is no evident lump.

YOU REALLY NEED TO KNOW

◆ Non-invasive cancer is called "carcinoma in situ." This type of cancer is limited to a duct or lobule.

◆ "Invasive carcinoma" is cancer that has spread into the surrounding breast tissue and can spread to other parts of the body.

◆ There are two main types of invasive breast cancer. The most common begins in the cells lining the ducts and is called "invasive ductal carcinoma." Invasive cancer arising from the lobules is called "invasive lobular carcinoma."

TYPES AND SITES OF BREAST CANCER

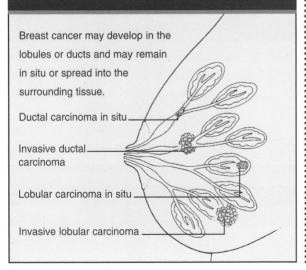

Breast cancer may develop in the lobules or ducts and may remain in situ or spread into the surrounding tissue.

Ductal carcinoma in situ

Invasive ductal carcinoma

Lobular carcinoma in situ

Invasive lobular carcinoma

Types of breast cancer

Types of breast cancer

If breast cancer is detected before it has spread to the lymph nodes in the armpit, there is a good chance that treatment will be successful.

How breast cancer spreads

If an invasive cancer has spread from the duct or lobe where it began into the surrounding breast tissue, this is called "local spread." Local spread may take place over many years, or more quickly. As the number of cancer cells increases, they form a lump (tumor). The tumor keeps growing and at some point will be big enough to be felt in the breast tissue. The size of the tumor when it is first detected is important when deciding on treatment.

In slightly less than two-thirds of cases, breast cancer does not spread beyond the breast and in many cases may be cured by surgery (with or without radiation therapy).

WHERE SECONDARY TUMORS ARE FOUND

Breast cancer probably spreads through the body in the bloodstream. If it does, secondary tumors (metastases) develop. These are usually in the bones, the spinal cord, lungs, liver, ovaries, or brain. For a few women, symptoms from the secondary tumor, such as bone pain, are the first indicators of their breast cancer.

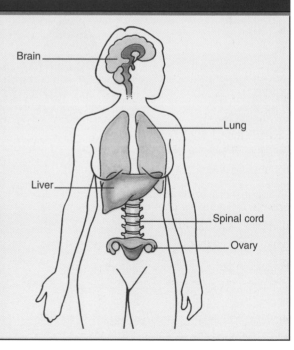

Brain

Lung

Liver

Spinal cord

Ovary

How secondary tumors develop

With any type of cancer, the first lump that forms is called the primary tumor. In breast cancer, most primary tumors are found in the upper, outer part of the breast. From here, the cancer may spread to form tumors in more distant parts of the body. These are called secondary tumors (or metastases).

Cancer is probably spread by the bloodstream, although we are not yet certain exactly how. We do know that the lymph nodes in the armpit act as signals (or markers) as to how likely a particular breast cancer is to spread. This is why you should examine your armpits as well as your breasts during breast self-examination (see p. 27) to try to detect any nodes that may be affected. Affected lymph nodes become swollen and enlarged.

If the lymph nodes are not affected, the chance of the cancer spreading is relatively low. If the lymph nodes are affected, the chance of the cancer spreading is higher, although the cancer almost certainly does not spread from the lymph nodes themselves.

Where does it spread to?

Once cancer cells have spread from the breast to other sites in the body, they start to grow, forming the secondary tumors. If it does spread, breast cancer most commonly spreads to bones, the liver, or lungs, and sometimes to other places such as the ovaries, the spinal cord, or the brain.

Because of the possibility of the cancer spreading, cancer treatment often includes chemotherapy (see p. 54). Chemotherapy is used to try and destroy all cancer cells in the whole body, not just those in the breast.

**YOU REALLY
NEED TO KNOW**

◆ Local spread is when the tumor spreads into the surrounding healthy breast tissue.

◆ Distant spread to other parts of the body is called metastasis. Breast cancer cells may spread to the bones, lungs, liver, ovaries, spinal cord, or brain. The tumors that grow at these sites are called secondary tumors or metastases.

Types of breast cancer

Breast cancer research

✓ It can make you anxious to be told that there are different ways of treating your breast cancer. Make sure you have all the information you need.

✓ You may be invited to join a clinical trial. These trials are scientifically designed to try to find out more facts about a disease so new treatments can be developed. You do not have to take part, but you may choose to if you know what the purpose of the trial is.

Nowadays, it is relatively easy to diagnose breast cancer, but once the diagnosis is made things become less clear cut. There has been a lot of research on the subject, but it has not yet provided all the answers, and there are still many things we do not know about breast cancer.

Research into the causes

One of the most important discoveries in breast cancer research was finding two breast cancer genes in 1994 (see p. 17). Women in families who carry these genes have an increased tendency to develop breast cancer. Further research is needed to find out exactly how these genes work, and experts hope this will lead to a breakthrough in understanding and possibly preventing

COPING WITH THE DIAGNOSIS

◆ The diagnosis of breast cancer can cause feelings of shock, disbelief, fear, and anxiety. You are entitled to a second opinion, and you are likely to be referred to a breast cancer specialist.

◆ Once the diagnosis has been confirmed, finding out more about your disease will help you to make the right decisions. Take time to find out as much information as you need to help you make informed choices.

◆ You may be feeling anxious when you see the doctor, which will not help you to ask the right questions or remember the answers. Write questions down beforehand and take your partner or a friend with you, and take notes of what you are told, or bring a tape recorder with you.

breast cancer altogether. At least 90 percent of breast cancers, however, are not caused by these genes, and we still do not know exactly why the disease develops.

Research into the types

To predict how a cancer will behave and so decide on the best course of treatment, we need to know as much as possible about its nature. New tests to identify the exact type of cancer are currently being developed. These include looking at the cancer's sensitivity to hormones and measuring other markers that indicate how aggressive (likely to spread) it is.

Genetic markers (oncogenes) that appear to influence growth rate, and therefore outlook, have been found in some breast cancers. The most common is ERB-B2 (see p. 60). New therapies act directly on proteins produced by these oncogenes to interfere with the cancer's growth.

Research into the treatment

Because breast cancer includes a range of conditions, there are a number of treatment options (see p. 38). Doctors now try to save the breast by offering smaller operations and using other treatments in addition to surgery. There is still debate about the best combinations of treatment to use and when to use which treatment, so you may find that your treatment differs from that of someone else you know.

What you can do

Every woman has the right to decide how much she wants to know about her illness and to choose between the different treatments offered to her. Informing yourself of all the facts allows you to choose what is best for you.

YOU REALLY NEED TO KNOW

◆ The tests used to diagnose breast cancer are reliable and are available to all women in the developed world.

◆ Breast cancer patients also need help in dealing with the emotional impact of the diagnosis.

◆ Do not be rushed into making decisions about treatment. Take what time you need to make the right choice for you.

Breast cancer research

Chapter

2

DIAGNOSIS

Symptoms of cancer

✓ Benign cysts in the breast are more likely to cause discomfort or pain than cancer is.

✓ In a very rare form of cancer, inflammatory breast cancer, the whole breast suddenly becomes red and feels hot and swollen.

The way most women (or their partners) find a cancer in the breast is by feeling a lump. For many women the lump has not caused any symptoms and seems to have appeared quite suddenly. Lumps in the breast are very common, and nine out of ten are not cancer. But because of the risk of cancer, if you find a lump—with or without symptoms—you should see your doctor promptly (within a few days).

Most breast cancers do not cause any specific symptoms, so it is difficult for a woman to reliably distinguish a benign lump from a cancer. But there are a few symptoms that may suggest breast cancer.

Nipple symptoms

If a tumor grows near the nipple, it may make the nipple become inverted (drawn inward). If one or both of your nipples has been inverted since puberty and you can evert them (pull them outward), there is no need to worry. It is only when one nipple becomes inverted later in life and cannot be easily everted that there is reason to suspect cancer.

Occasionally breast cancer may cause bleeding from the nipple, or a rust-colored or bloodstained discharge. Most bleeding or discharge is caused by a benign condition, such as a cyst. Even so, if you notice a discharge, have it checked by your doctor.

Skin symptoms

Sometimes you may notice that skin over the lump seems to be attached to the lump when you move your arm. This is called tethering. Accumulation of fluid in the tissues of the skin may make the skin look pitted, rather like the peel of an orange.

BREAST SELF-EXAMINATION

Regular breast self-examination (BSE) helps you become familiar with your body so you will be able to spot changes.

1. Undress to the waist and stand in front of a mirror (left). With your arms loosely by your sides, look for any alteration in the shape, size, and symmetry of your breasts and nipples.

2. Raise your arms above your head and again check for changes. Turn sideways to see your breasts in profile (right).

3. Now put your hands on your hips and push downward, so your chest muscles tense up. Look again for any of the signs listed above.

4. The next part of BSE is better done lying down. With one arm behind your head, use the flat of your fingers to feel firmly for any lump or thickening.

5. Work your way around in a spiral, covering all areas of the breast (left). Remember also to check your armpits. It is important that your doctor follow the same steps when you go to the office. If you are not happy with the way your doctor examines you, ask for a second opinion, or bring it up for discussion.

YOU REALLY NEED TO KNOW

◆ Some women naturally have lumpier breasts than others. Breast self-examination makes you familiar with what is normal for you.

◆ Any change in your breast, nipple, or armpit needs to be examined by a doctor.

◆ Breast self-examination is best done once a month, at the end of your period, when the breasts are softer.

Symptoms of cancer

X-rays and scans

Mammography

When an X-ray of the breast is taken to be used to look for cancer, the process is called a mammography. The X-ray is called a mammogram. A mammogram can pick up very small tumors before they have spread into the surrounding breast tissue and lymph nodes, even before they can be felt as a lump.

In the U.S., breast cancer screening involves routine annual mammograms for women ages 40 and older. A routine mammography aims to pick up as many breast cancers as possible as early as possible. Younger women have denser breasts, which do not show up as well on a mammogram, so only those women who have a high risk of developing breast cancer are offered regular mammograms.

WHAT DOES A MAMMOGRAM SHOW?

A mammogram is a picture of the breast on X-ray film. Cancer shows up as a white lump, a group of little white specks, or a combination of the two. The results are not always absolutely clear—the radiologist may have difficulty interpreting the mammogram, or there may be an area that does not show up well. If this is the case, you may be asked to come back for another mammogram.

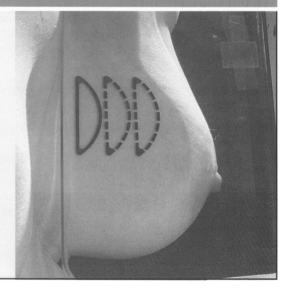

28

How is a mammogram done?

The nurse will ask you to undress to the waist, and wipe your breasts clean of any talcum powder or deodorant. The radiographer will then compress each breast in turn between lucite plates, one of which contains the X-ray film to take an X-ray. Your breasts need to be as flat as possible for a good-quality picture. A mammography must be done by a radiology technician and the results interpreted by a radiologist.

Many women find mammographies uncomfortable, and a few even find the process painful, but it helps if you are prepared and know what to expect in advance. Occasionally, your breasts may feel bruised for a few days afterward.

Ultrasound scan

An ultrasound scan is a picture created using sound waves instead of X-rays. It is not used routinely in screening for breast cancer because it is not as good at detecting cancer as a mammogram. However, it may be used as an extra test in some cases, to get as much information as possible about abnormalities seen on a mammogram. Ultrasound is good at picking up cysts, so it can be helpful for younger women (under 35) who have a lump that is most likely to be a cyst.

Magnetic resonance imaging (MRI)

Magnetic resonance imaging builds up a computerized picture from the way the body's tissues bounce back magnetic waves. Researchers are currently looking at how an MRI may best be used to detect breast cancer. It may also be able to tell us about the type of cancer and help predict its behavior.

YOU REALLY NEED TO KNOW

◆ If you are over 40, you should have a mammogram annually.

◆ Most breast cancers show up on a mammogram, even very early in the disease.

◆ Ultrasound is not used as a screening test for breast cancer because fewer than half of all breast cancers can be seen on the scan.

X-rays and scans

Cytology and biopsy

✗ Fine needle aspiration cytology takes a sample of individual cells, but cannot show if a tumor is invasive or in situ.

✓ A biopsy sample contains a group of cells joined together, so it is possible to tell whether the cancer cells have spread from the lobule or duct into the surrounding tissue.

✓ Some radiologists may perform fine needle aspiration cytology and biopsy on the same day.

Cytology

All suspicious breast lumps found during a mammogram must be examined more closely. A pathologist looks at cells from the lump under a microscope (this is called cytology) to see whether or not they are malignant. Cancer cells look different from normal cells.

Fine needle aspiration cytology

In fine needle aspiration cytology (FNAC), cells are withdrawn using a thin needle. With very small lumps, the specialist may use ultrasound or an X-ray to make sure the needle is in the right place. FNAC can show whether an area is a solid lump or a cyst—if it is a cyst, fluid will be drawn off and the cyst will collapse. Fluid from a cyst can be sent for analysis to make sure there are no cancer cells in it.

Aspiration is usually done without anesthetic, so you will feel the needle going in. As with most injections, the skin is the most sensitive part, and the aspiration itself is not painful. Asking questions and discussing your fears can help to make the procedure less stressful. There may be some internal bleeding, and your breast may feel tender and bruised for a few days. The bruising may be enough to show up on X-ray, so mammograms are always done before fine needle aspiration.

An aspiration takes only a few minutes. You may get the results the same day, or your doctor may call in a few days. If the result shows abnormal cells, the next step is a biopsy.

Biopsy

In a needle biopsy (also called a core biopsy, mammotome, or a tru-cut biopsy), a piece of tissue about an inch long and the diameter of a pencil lead is removed under local anesthetic, using a thicker needle than the one used for FNAC. If the suspicious area is small, the biopsy may be done under X-ray guidance to make sure the right area is sampled. The pathologist then cuts the tissue into thin slices and examines them under the microscope. It is a bigger, slightly more invasive procedure than FNAC. Applying pressure or ice to the site once the needle has been removed will help to reduce bruising.

If there is any doubt about the diagnosis after mammography, FNAC, and core biopsy, an open biopsy may prove helpful. This is a larger version of needle biopsy, done in the hospital under general anesthetic. If the whole lump and some surrounding tissue are removed, this is called an excisional biopsy or lumpectomy.

YOU REALLY NEED TO KNOW

◆ Cells taken from a breast lump are examined under a microscope. Cancer cells look different from normal cells.

◆ Fine needle aspiration and biopsies are always done by experienced professionals.

◆ Fine needle aspiration and needle biopsies may be uncomfortable and cause some bruising and internal bleeding, but they are not usually painful.

FINE NEEDLE ASPIRATION

After cleaning the skin, the doctor (a gynecologist, radiologist, or breast surgeon) holds the lump firmly and inserts a fine needle into it, rather like giving an injection. He or she draws out (aspirates) some of the cells into a syringe before taking the needle out and smearing the cells on to a slide. The cells are then examined under a microscope.

Cytology and biopsy

Chapter

3

TREATMENT
& CARE

What influences treatment?

✓ Different cancers respond in different ways, so some treatments are more effective than others.

✓ Tests and investigations help the doctor to choose the most effective treatment.

Each type of breast cancer behaves in a different manner. But there are two crucial questions in deciding which treatment is best in each particular case. First, is the chance of distant spreading (spreading to other parts of the body) high or low? And second, what can be done to reduce that chance?

How doctors predict spreading

The chance of distant spreading will influence your doctor's recommendations and your choice of treatment options. If your cancer has a high chance of spreading to other parts of your body, and if a treatment can reduce that chance, your doctor will recommend that treatment more strongly—and you may be more likely to accept it. If the chance of the cancer spreading is low, you may be less motivated to accept a particular treatment.

PREDICTING THE CHANCE OF SPREAD

These factors all help to predict the chance that breast cancer will spread:

◆ Whether the tumor has spread to the lymph nodes in the armpit, and if so how many lymph nodes are involved.

◆ The size of the original tumor. This refers to the size as measured when it has been removed—the apparent size before the operation may be misleading.

◆ Laboratory tests on the tumor for hormone receptors. These tests are not always done, particularly if the original tumor was very small.

◆ Other tests, including tests on the blood, that are done in some cases.

Doctors cannot tell every woman with breast cancer whether her particular cancer will spread or not, but they can give some estimate as to whether the chance of spreading is high or low. Three features are routinely used to help in that prediction: whether the cancer has spread to the lymph nodes in the armpit, and if so how many of them are affected; the size of the tumor; and whether the tumor is producing hormone receptors.

Tests you may be offered include a chest X-ray, a blood test, to see if the liver is involved, and a bone scan to show any "hot spots" where tumor cells may be growing. Other possible options include tests to show how many cells are actually multiplying at the time and any invasion into the lymph vessels. A blood test may also be done to measure substances called CEA, CA 15-3, CA 19-9, and others, as rising levels may indicate that the cancer is recurring or spreading.

Can the outcome be predicted?

It is very difficult to say with certainty what the outcome of a particular treatment will be for a particular individual. For example, comparing figures from two studies may suggest that one form of treatment has a higher survival rate after five years than the other. But the first study may have involved far fewer women and, if repeated on a larger scale, could prove to have a much lower survival rate. Because of this uncertainty, you should try not to rely on information from an impersonal source, such as TV, newspapers, or magazines. You need to get your information from someone who can explain what any statistics mean in your case and can talk through your treatment options with you, answering any questions you may have.

What influences treatment?

The holistic approach

✓ It is your doctor's duty to inform you about treatment options, what to expect, and any side effects and risks involved.

✓ In order to play an active role in your treatment, you need to be able to make informed decisions— the experts are there to guide, give advice, and answer all your questions.

✓ If you want to see a particular specialist, for example a psychologist, and your team does not include one, you can ask for a referral.

Medical staff are now aware of the need to consider the person as a whole, rather than just deal with her disease. The medical team looks at the emotional, social, spiritual, and financial aspects of treatment as well as the physical.

All patients are entitled to the best possible treatment. For women with breast cancer, this starts with diagnosis. If there is a possibility that you have breast cancer, your

A TEAM APPROACH TO BREAST CANCER

You will be treated by a team of professionals, including some or all of the following:

INTERNIST OR GYNECOLOGIST
Usually arranges the first referral to a breast specialist.

ONCOLOGIST
A cancer specialist who advises on overall treatment. A radiation oncologist is trained in giving radiation therapy; a medical oncologist gives chemotherapy only.

RADIOLOGIST
A doctor specializing in the study of X-rays and other imaging techniques. He or she will interpret your mammogram.

PATHOLOGIST
A doctor specializing in the effect of disease on body tissues, and how cells look under the microscope.

X-RAY TECHNICIAN
Trained to use X-ray machines.

3

doctor needs to arrange a timely referral to a breast surgeon. At certain breast cancer centers, you may get a confirmed diagnosis in one day. Even when you need to wait for a firm diagnosis, there is no need to make any decisions about treatment until you know for sure what your diagnosis is. In most cases, up to three weeks delay in starting treatment will not alter its effectiveness.

BREAST SURGEON

A surgery specialist who performs breast biopsies, excisional biopsies, lumpectomy, mastectomy, and reconstruction.

ONCOLOGY NURSE

Nurse with training in dealing with breast disease and other tumors. Tells you what to expect and gives support and advice.

FLOOR NURSE

Cares for you when you are in the hospital.

PHYSICAL THERAPIST

Gives you exercises to do after surgery.

PSYCHOLOGIST

Professional counseling can help you to deal with decisions about treatment, depression and anxiety, and family issues.

SOCIAL WORKER

Can help solve practical difficulties, including transportation, childcare, and financial issues.

YOU REALLY NEED TO KNOW

◆ Your whole life changes when you are diagnosed with a life-threatening disease such as breast cancer, and the care you receive needs to address as many of your needs as possible.

◆ Breast lumps that might be cancer need to be investigated urgently, i.e. within three weeks.

◆ You have the right to ask for a second opinion, and you do not have to make any decisions until the diagnosis is definite.

The holistic approach

Principles of treatment

Treating breast cancer has three aims: to remove the primary tumor, to reduce the chance that the cancer will return in the breast or the armpit (local recurrence), and to reduce the chance that cancer will spread and establish metastases elsewhere in the body.

Local treatment consists of surgery and radiation therapy. It is aimed at the lump and the lymph nodes in the armpit. Treatment additional to surgery is called adjuvant therapy, and consists of combinations of radiation therapy, chemotherapy, and hormone therapy. Chemotherapy and hormone therapy are also called systemic treatment, because they affect the whole body, not just the local area, killing any cancer cells that have spread to sites beyond the breast and armpit (axilla). Even when there is no obvious distant spreading, there may be micrometastasis, which is spreading that is too small to be detected.

Your treatment plan

The treatment you receive will depend on your diagnosis. You may be offered a choice of operations, a combination of surgery and radiation therapy, or a combination of surgery and systemic treatment.

For women with early invasive breast cancer, the survival rate has been shown to be the same with either breast conservation or modified radical mastectomy (see p. 42). Breast conservation, which consists of lumpectomy (removal of the lump only), axillary node dissection, and radiation therapy, can be considered whatever your age. But it is not suitable for women who choose not to have radiation therapy or who prefer to have the whole breast removed for peace of mind.

Most treatments for advanced cancer involving the skin and muscles of the armpit, with or without

TYPES OF THERAPY

LOCAL TREATMENT	◆ surgery ◆ radiation therapy (RT)
ADJUVANT THERAPY	◆ RT (local) ◆ chemotherapy (systemic) ◆ hormone therapy (systemic)
LOCAL TREATMENT WITH ADJUVANT THERAPY	◆ surgery + RT
SYSTEMIC TREATMENT (ALMOST ALWAYS INCLUDES SURGERY)	◆ surgery + chemotherapy ◆ RT + chemotherapy ◆ surgery + RT + chemotherapy ◆ surgery + hormone therapy ◆ surgery + hormone therapy + chemotherapy ◆ surgery + RT + hormone therapy ◆ surgery + RT + chemotherapy + hormone therapy

YOU REALLY NEED TO KNOW

◆ Treatment is aimed at the breast lump, the lymph nodes, and distant disease.

◆ The most likely treatment for early breast cancer is surgery to remove the primary tumor.

◆ Treatment can be any combination of surgery, radiation therapy, chemotherapy, or hormone therapy.

metastatic spread, include systemic therapy. For pre-menopausal women, this is usually chemotherapy and for older women it is commonly hormone therapy.

Principles of treatment

Surgical treatment

✓ Lumpectomy is a good option for some women, who often make a quicker recovery than those who have a mastectomy.

✗ Lumpectomy is not a good choice for women with very large tumors, as it would leave one breast much smaller than the other.

✓ If lumpectomy is not an option for you, you will be offered a mastectomy.

Surgery aims to remove as much cancerous tissue as possible from the breast. It is usually the first treatment for breast cancer, and most women will have at least one operation during the course of their disease.

Lumpectomy

Studies have shown that for smaller tumors, a less extensive operation that removes the tumor but leaves most of the remaining breast tissue intact is as effective as removing the entire breast. Surgery that saves part of the breast is described as conservative, and although it is not suitable in all cases, many women have been spared the trauma of losing a breast.

In a lumpectomy, also called a partial mastectomy, the surgeon removes the lump plus a margin of breast tissue around it. The tissue that has been removed is sent to the laboratory where it is examined to check that the margins are clear of cancer. The operation is done under general anesthetic, and you may be able to go

Depending on breast size, and the size and site of the tumor, the cosmetic result of lumpectomy can be very good.

home the same day. If not, you will only be in the hospital for a few days. There will be a small scar where the incision was made, and you will have stitches, possibly a tube to drain blood and fluids, and a dressing, which will be removed once healing is under way.

If the tumor lies directly below the nipple, lumpectomy includes removal of both the nipple and the areola, which leaves the breast mound but no nipple. If there is more than one tumor in the breast, or if the tumor is quite advanced, conservative surgery is not an option for you.

In most cases, the lymph nodes in the armpit have to be sampled through a separate incision, so if you have a lumpectomy, you will usually require two incisions. You should receive RT to the breast (and sometimes also to the armpit) to reduce the chance of local recurrence.

Radical mastectomy

An operation in which the whole breast is removed is called a mastectomy, and there are three different types. The oldest is called radical mastectomy, but is hardly ever used now. Radical mastectomy—which is, as its name suggests, the most extensive form of mastectomy—involves removal of the entire breast including the skin and nipple, the nodes from the armpit, and the fat and muscles of the chest wall (the pectoralis muscles). This leaves only the rib cage covered by skin, and a very long scar. It weakens the arm because some of the muscles are removed. If you are offered a radical mastectomy, you may want to ask for a second opinion because advances in treatment mean it is rarely necessary to have such a major operation.

YOU REALLY NEED TO KNOW

◆ Surgery is usually the first treatment for breast cancer. Most women will have at least one operation during the course of their disease.

◆ Surgery that saves part of the breast is called conservative. It is not suitable for women with very large tumors or more than one tumor in the breast.

◆ Mastectomy is removal of the entire breast. There are three types, which differ in the amount of muscle and the number of lymph nodes removed.

Surgical treatment

Surgical treatment

Modified radical mastectomy

This is less extensive and less mutilating than radical mastectomy. The breast, some of the lymph nodes, and the smaller of the two chest muscles are removed. It leaves the pectoralis major muscle, which gives a better shape to the chest, and allows normal arm movement. Modified radical mastectomy is very commonly used in treating breast cancer.

Simple mastectomy

Simple mastectomy, also called total mastectomy, involves removal of the breast alone. It does not always include axillary node dissection, although some nodes may be removed to look for cancer (sentinel node sampling). The chest muscles are not removed.

What to expect

Mastectomy is a major operation, and you will be in the hospital for between five and ten days. After the operation you will feel tender and bruised around the

It can be very helpful to talk to someone who has been through breast surgery before finally deciding on the best treatment for you.

wound, and your shoulder might feel stiff. During some mastectomies, the surgeon inserts a drain. This is a small tube to remove fluid that may otherwise collect behind the stitches. The drain is usually removed between three and five days after the operation. Your stitches may be taken out while you are still in the hospital, or you may have to go back to have them removed.

Deciding on surgery

Before deciding on surgery, make sure you know all the facts. Discuss your options with your oncologist and other members of the team. Find out if the hospital can put you in touch with another breast cancer patient, or contact one of the voluntary organizations (see p. 78). Talking to someone who has been through breast surgery may help you to decide what is best for you. This is a good stage to talk about your options after the operation because what you choose now can limit your choices later. When deciding what type of surgery is best, you and your doctor need to go through the implications for reconstruction (see p. 48) and adjuvant therapy (see p. 50).

Sentinel node sampling

Surgery to the axilla (see p. 44) can increase the risk of the operation, but because it is important to know whether the lymph nodes contain cancer or not, a procedure called "sentinel node biopsy" is sometimes carried out. During initial breast surgery, a radioactive dye is injected into the lymphatic vessels that lead to the axilla. The first node found to contain dye is removed and immediately examined under a microscope. If it is negative for cancer, no further surgery is required in this area, but if it is positive more nodes need to be removed.

YOU REALLY NEED TO KNOW

◆ You need time and support, in the form of advice and counseling, before making a final decision on the type of operation.

◆ It is important to be fully informed of all the advantages and disadvantages of the options open to you.

◆ Talk about reconstructive surgery with your doctor before you decide to go ahead with any operation.

Surgical treatment

Surgical treatment

✓ Treating the axilla does not prevent breast cancer from spreading, but it is important in controlling local disease.

✗ A diagnosis of breast cancer during pregnancy does not always mean the pregnancy must be terminated.

✓ Some types of chemotherapy can be given in the last three months of pregnancy for the treatment of advanced, aggressive breast cancer.

✗ Hormone therapy is never offered to pregnant women who have breast cancer.

Treating the axilla

Removing the lymph nodes of the axilla (armpit) makes it possible to see exactly how many are involved, and at what level. If most of the lymph nodes are involved, there is a higher chance of the cancer growing back in the armpit after surgery. This is called local recurrence and is difficult to treat. Up to 40 percent of women with invasive breast cancer have affected axillary nodes.

Axillary nodes are removed as part of a mastectomy. If they are removed as part of a lumpectomy, the surgeon makes a separate incision to remove them. In some cases, the surgeon carries out sentinel node dissection (see p. 43) so he or she does not have to remove a large number of nodes unnecessarily. Removing the nodes doesn't stop the cancer from spreading, but it does help to control the cancer in the axillary area.

REMOVING THE AXILLARY NODES

Axillary nodes are usually removed as part of a mastectomy. In axillary node dissection, all the nodes are removed. If only a few are removed to see if cancer is present, it is called sampling.

Nodes

Results of axillary surgery

Apart from the surgical scars, there is usually very little physical change after surgery. Sometimes, the skin of the armpit and the inside of the arm gets numb or tingly, and the arm on that side may swell as a result of fluid build up (or lymphedema, see p. 47). This is more likely if all the nodes are removed, or if you have a combination of surgery and radiation therapy to the axilla.

BREAST CANCER IN PREGNANCY

◆ Breast cancer occurs in 1 pregnancy in every 3,000. The diagnosis is made in the usual way, although the normal breast changes in pregnancy may make feeling a lump more difficult. Because of the possible effects on the developing fetus, treatment is slightly different.

◆ The standard treatment is modified radical mastectomy with lymph node dissection. Conservative treatment is not offered because radiation can harm the developing fetus, and the chance of the cancer recurring in lumpectomy without radiotherapy is up to 40 percent.

◆ If the diagnosis is made in the last three months, there are more options. If the pregnancy is near term, treatment may be delayed by a few weeks to deliver a term baby. If there are several months remaining, management of the pregnancy may be determined following consultation with an obstetrician, breast surgeon, and oncologist. Chemotherapy may be given safely in the second and third trimester (4th-9th months) without increases in the risk of birth defects, stillbirths, prematurity, or low birth weight.

3

YOU REALLY NEED TO KNOW

◆ If the axillary lymph nodes are involved, you will need treatment to this area.

◆ Removing all the involved lymph nodes from the axilla reduces the chance of local recurrence.

◆ Pregnant women who have breast cancer do not have to terminate the pregnancy, but in some cases delivery may be induced early.

◆ The type of treatment offered to a pregnant woman who has breast cancer depends on the stage of her pregnancy, the size of the tumor, and on some of the characteristics of the tumor cells.

Surgical treatment

Surgical treatment

Bringing something comforting like a photo can help you feel better in hospital.

Make sure you have some change handy for small purchases and a phonecard for phone calls. Mobile phones are not usually allowed.

In the hospital

You will be admitted to the hospital the day before or early on the day of your operation. The nursing staff will ask questions about your lifestyle and health, weigh you, and take your temperature and blood pressure. You will also be seen by a doctor and you may be able to talk to the anesthesiologist.

By the time you are admitted, you should know exactly what operation you are going to have, but you will still need to sign a consent form giving your permission for the surgery. As the doctor goes through the consent form, ask about anything you do not understand.

You will be asked not to eat or drink anything from around midnight the night before your operation to reduce the chance of vomiting or choking while you are under anesthesia. You should not see, hear, or feel anything while you are under general anesthesia, and

WHY YOU NEED AN IV

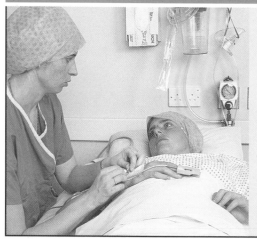

Soon after you are admitted to the hospital for your operation, the doctor will insert an intravenous catheter (also called an IV tube) into a vein in your arm or hand. This will be used for giving you fluids and medication after your operation, so you do not need to have repeated injections. The IV will be left in place until you are well enough to eat and drink again.

you will not remember anything when you wake up, although you may feel drowsy and confused. The nursing staff can give you something if you feel sick.

After the operation

You will be encouraged to get out of bed as soon as possible. There is no need to be in any pain, so ask for painkillers if you find you need them. At first, your arm movement will be restricted, but you will be given exercises to do to help this. Drains are usually taken out after three to five days and stitches within two weeks. The scar will heal in two to four weeks, and will fade in time.

Lymphedema

After surgery to the lymph nodes or radiation therapy to the axilla, the flow of lymph may be blocked, and this can cause the arm to swell up (lymphedema). Improved techniques have made this less common, but it does still occur, especially after extensive axillary surgery or a combination of surgery and radiation therapy to the axilla. Treatment includes massage to encourage lymph drainage, use of a mechanical pump to reduce swelling, exercise, and raising the arm.

Other complications

The wound may feel hot for a couple of days. If it becomes infected, it will be red and tender, and you may need antibiotics. If fluid builds up behind the stitches after the drain has been removed or if one was not used, it may need to be drained. Other complications that can occur after any operation are chest infection and a clot in a leg vein. Both can be prevented, or treated if they appear, but occasionally they can be serious.

3

Surgical treatment

Reconstructive surgery

✓ You can have a nipple reconstructed surgically, using skin taken from behind your ear or from your inner thigh.

✓ Paste-on nipples are available from special supply shops.

✓ A nipple and areola can be tattooed onto the breast mound.

After a mastectomy, it is often possible to reconstruct the breast area to restore the contour and original appearance of the breast. No reconstruction will ever look or feel exactly like the natural breast, but using tissue from your own body, or a synthetic implant, the surgeon can create a breast that looks fine except under very close examination. Not all women want reconstruction, but if you think that it might make you feel more positive, ask if it is available in your case. It is not suitable for women with very advanced disease, nor for those whose cancer is actively spreading.

When is reconstruction done?

Reconstructive surgery can be done immediately (at the time the natural breast is removed), or later, when other treatment is completed. Some doctors prefer to wait for

DURING A BREAST IMPLANT

The doctor inserts a temporary expanding implant under the mastectomy scar (there is no need for a second scar). Each week he or she injects more fluid into the implant and the skin gradually stretches (expands) until there is enough space underneath to insert the permanent implant. The permanent implant is made of silicone filled with saline fluid or silicone gel. The end result can look and feel very natural, but there is a risk of your body reacting to the foreign material, causing a buildup of fibrous tissue that makes the breast feel hard. The other disadvantages are that it is done in stages, takes time, and requires weekly visits. There is also a chance that the implant may leak.

two years, because reconstruction can make it harder to detect any recurrence. The advantages of immediate reconstruction are that you need only one major operation, and therefore only one general anesthetic. Some women also find it less traumatic to wake up with a breast mound already in place. The disadvantages are that the operation itself takes longer to perform than mastectomy alone, and there is a slight increase in the number of complications that may occur, which may mean delaying further treatment.

Waiting until all local and adjuvant therapy (see p. 50) is completed makes sense to many women. Another advantage is that it gives you time to adjust to your new, altered body appearance, to consider all your options, and to explore alternatives to surgery.

Different types of reconstruction

Reconstructive surgery cannot create a perfect replacement in a single operation. The new breast will look different, and it usually takes a couple of more minor operations to complete. The surgeon can either use tissue from your own body (autologous tissue) or an implant. Suitable tissue can be taken from the muscles of the back, stomach, buttocks, or outside of the thigh. When using the back or stomach muscle, the surgeon cuts a flap of tissue, still attached to its original blood supply, and sews it into place over the mastectomy site. The back muscle has a good blood supply, but leaves a visible scar and is not large enough to fill more than a C-cup bra. It also limits arm and shoulder movement. The stomach muscle has more tissue available, but may not be suitable if you are overweight since it weakens the stomach wall and can lead to a hernia.

YOU REALLY NEED TO KNOW

◆ Reconstructive surgery can be done at the same time as a mastectomy.

◆ Choosing delayed reconstruction gives you time to adjust to your new shape, and to consider all of your possible options.

◆ The surgeon can reconstruct the breast using tissue taken from your own body, especially back or stomach muscles.

◆ Breast implants can give very good results, but some women's bodies do not accept the silicone that is used in implants.

Reconstructive surgery

Adjuvant treatment

The real problem with breast cancer is that, even after an operation, it can recur in the breast and can also spread to other parts of the body, where it forms secondary tumors. Treatment that is given after surgery to reduce the chance of the cancer spreading is called adjuvant treatment. Even when there is no evidence of local spread, the seeds of distant spread may be present but undetectable. Adjuvant treatment aims to eradicate these seeds so no secondary cancers develop. Since this is not always a realistic goal, the second aim is to delay recurrence of the cancer. Adjuvant therapy may take the form of radiation therapy, chemotherapy, or hormone therapy.

Who has adjuvant treatment?

As with most aspects of this complex disease, there is no simple answer as to who should have adjuvant treatment. When deciding whether or not to give it, doctors try to predict the likelihood that the patient's tumor will recur. It is impossible to know for sure how a cancer will behave, but there are some factors that indicate that recurrence or distant spreading is more likely. These include the invasiveness of the tumor (in situ tumors do not need adjuvant therapy), the size of the tumor, the number of lymph nodes involved, whether the tumor is sensitive to the hormones estrogen and progesterone (measured using hormone receptor tests), and the aggressiveness of the tumor.

Which type of therapy?

The exact type of adjuvant therapy recommended will depend on three things—whether you have had your menopause or are still having periods, whether the

NEOADJUVANT THERAPY

Therapy can be used to shrink a cancer before surgery. This is known as neoadjuvant therapy. It makes surgery technically easier and perhaps more effective. Also, giving therapy such as chemotherapy before surgery can show whether or not the cancer responds to those drugs. If so, they may be useful after the operation as well.

tumor had hormone receptors on it when it was tested, and, when there is more than one option to be considered, your own feelings and preferences.

Radiation therapy (RT)

In radiation therapy, high-energy radiation (similar to X-rays) is used to treat disease. When radiation therapy is used to treat breast cancer, it consists of directing beams of radiation at the cancer site to kill any cancer cells left behind after surgery. In the past, all women with breast cancer used to receive radiation therapy, but doctors now select those who will benefit most to avoid irradiating women unnecessarily.

When is radiation therapy given?

Conservative therapy for early disease consists of radiation therapy given after lumpectomy and axillary node dissection. This gives the same results as modified radical mastectomy. In more advanced cancer, when the tumor is larger, or there is node involvement or the cancer has spread to the skin and chest wall, radiation therapy is given after mastectomy and axillary dissection.

YOU REALLY NEED TO KNOW

◆ Chemotherapy, radiation therapy, and hormone therapy are the most commonly used types of adjuvant therapy.

◆ Adjuvant therapy has its own risks and side effects.

◆ In situ cancer does not need treatment with adjuvant therapy.

Adjuvant treatment

Adjuvant treatment

Where is the radiation directed?

After a lumpectomy, the radiation therapy will be directed at the remaining breast tissue. With modern techniques, it is possible to limit the amount of radiation that reaches the ribs, lungs, and heart, although small doses will pass through healthy tissue on the way to the cancer site. After a mastectomy, the chest wall will be irradiated, and if there is node involvement or a strong chance that the cancer will recur, the axilla will also be treated, as will the area above the collarbone, where other lymph nodes are situated.

Radiation therapy is also used to treat local recurrence at the original site or in the armpit, and in late-stage breast cancer to try to shrink a tumor that is too big to remove.

How is radiation therapy given?

An average course of radiation therapy consists of treatment five days a week for five or six weeks, starting approximately a month after surgery, when you are able

To make sure you receive the right dose of radiation in the correct place, you have to lie in the same position each time (usually lying down with your arm above your head). You need to lie absolutely still while the radiation is being given.

to move your arm and shoulder again. You will go to the hospital each day and return home afterward. Treatment takes a few minutes—the actual exposure to radiation lasts only about five minutes, but it also takes a little while to position you correctly.

Side effects of radiation therapy

While you are having treatment, you may feel very tired, but you will not lose the hair on your head and you are unlikely to feel nauseous. The main short-term side effect is a skin reaction. The area may feel "sunburned," and become dry and scaly or itchy. The skin often turns darker, but this is not permanent. You may also get some little red marks caused by small blood vessels bursting.

You can try to prevent problems by careful skin care. This includes gentle washing, avoiding the use of soap, talcum powder, and skin lotion, and not exposing the area to the sun. You may be given a mild steroid cream or a petroleum jelly dressing to apply. Most skin reactions settle within a few weeks of the end of treatment.

The long-term side effects of radiation therapy are more troublesome, but are rare. Approximately 12 percent of women who have axillary surgery and radiation therapy develop lymphedema, or swelling of the arm (see p. 47). Tell your doctor if you notice any puffiness or swelling so it can be treated as soon as possible.

Occasionally, radiation therapy affects the surrounding healthy tissues. This can lead to problems such as pneumonitis, which is an inflammation of the lungs. It is very rare, but if it does develop, it causes shortness of breath and a dry cough. Another possible problem is damage to the ribs, which may be weakened by radiation therapy and, quite possibly, can break.

3

YOU REALLY NEED TO KNOW

◆ Radiation therapy kills cancer cells with high-energy radiation.

◆ Not everybody who has breast cancer needs radiation therapy.

◆ Radiation therapy has few side effects, compared with chemotherapy.

Adjuvant treatment

Systemic therapy

Systemic therapy is treatment that circulates throughout the whole body looking for cancer cells. It aims to improve the survival rate in women whose cancer has already spread beyond the primary tumor.

If you have been through menopause and your cancer has hormone receptors, hormone therapy is generally recommended. If it had no hormone receptors, chemotherapy is usually recommended. Premenopausal women are usually recommended to have chemotherapy.

Chemotherapy

Treatment of cancer with cytotoxic drugs (drugs designed to find and destroy cancer cells) is known as chemotherapy. Side effects occur because some healthy cells are sacrificed along the way. Cancer drugs need to be toxic to be effective, but those that are generally used for breast cancer are some of the least harmful.

In premenopausal women, the most common type of chemotherapy is a combination of three drugs—

DRUGS USED IN CHEMOTHERAPY

First-line drugs in current use in chemotherapy treatment for breast cancer include:

◆ Adriamycin (doxorubicin)

◆ Cyclophosphamide (cisplatin)

◆ Methotrexate

◆ Fluoruoracil

◆ Epirubicin

◆ Paclitaxel (taxol)

Of patients who do not respond to first-line drugs, between 23 and 30 percent will respond to second-line combinations of drugs, of which there are many in current use.

cyclophosphamide, methotrexate, and 5-fluoruoracil (CMF). The cyclophosphamide is usually given as a tablet daily for a few days; the other two drugs are given through an IV inserted into your arm (see p. 46). If you have an IV, you may need to stay in the hospital overnight, but usually you can have your chemotherapy as an out-patient.

Postmenopausal women with tumors negative for hormone receptors (see p. 58) are usually given a different chemotherapy, which contains a drug called adriamycin.

The timing of chemotherapy varies, but it is usually given for six months in total (four for adriamycin-containing combinations), with a series of treatments once a month. Traditionally, chemotherapy was given after surgery and radiation therapy, but ongoing research is looking at alternatives, such as giving half the chemotherapy, pausing for radiation therapy, then completing the treatment with more chemotherapy.

Very high-dose chemotherapy

Some cancers may respond to very high-dose chemotherapy, and if this is the case, you may be offered a bone marrow transplant. This means that some of your bone marrow will be removed before the chemotherapy starts, stored for you and then put back after chemotherapy. The same can be done with stem cells (the immature cells that divide to make new blood cells). Stem cells can be harvested from the blood or bone marrow, and because they have not been affected by the chemotherapy, when they are returned to the body they can still produce healthy blood cells. Whether this treatment is beneficial in breast cancer is still under review, so do discuss it with your doctor.

YOU REALLY NEED TO KNOW

◆ Systemic treatment is aimed at preventing or halting the growth of metastatic disease—that is, cancer that has spread to other parts of the body.

◆ All breast cancers with lymph node involvement need adjuvant therapy of some sort.

◆ Late stage cancer may be treated with palliative chemotherapy only. This relieves the pain and slows progress of the disease but does not cure the cancer.

Systemic therapy

Systemic therapy

✓ New treatments have made nausea and vomiting much less of a problem than they used to be.

✓ Mouth ulcers and infections can be prevented by careful brushing of the teeth and regular use of a mouthwash.

Side effects of chemotherapy

The most dangerous side effect is temporary suppression of the immune system, a serious problem for about 1 in 20 women. It occurs because the chemotherapy damages the bone marrow where the blood cells are made. If you do not have enough white cells, you cannot fight infection, so your blood will be tested before each treatment; and if your white cell count is too low, your chemotherapy dose will be adjusted or delayed. Red blood cells are also affected, and you may need a transfusion to raise your count.

Nausea and vomiting are very common. If this happens, future doses will be reduced as much as possible without interfering with their effectiveness. There are also new, effective treatments to prevent nausea. Chemotherapy leaves most people feeling drained, but energy levels usually return to normal about a month after the end of chemotherapy.

Some women also find they put on weight. Get advice on modifying your diet, and, if you feel up to it, join an enjoyable exercise program to help you feel better and prevent you from gaining weight.

Fertility problems

With chemotherapy, your periods can become irregular or stop. In younger women, menstruation tends to start again once treatment has ended, but about 40 percent of women will not menstruate again. After the age of 40, you are more likely to become infertile after chemotherapy. Some women experience menopausal symptoms, such as vaginal dryness and hot flushes. Simple lubricants may help with vaginal dryness, while hot flushes tend to disappear after a while.

LOSING YOUR HAIR

Hair loss is a distressing side effect that begins about three weeks after the start of chemotherapy. Not everybody loses all their hair, and you may find yours only gets thinner. The psychological effect of losing your hair can be traumatic, especially after losing a breast, but knowing it is not permanent and preparing for it in advance by buying a wig (see p. 67) helps many women cope better.

Preparing for chemotherapy

All these unpleasant possibilities, combined with the stress of having cancer, can be taxing emotionally and psychologically. You can prepare for the physical strain by getting plenty of rest, eating well, and taking vitamin and mineral supplements.

Emotionally you may find it helps to take the initiative and to think of chemotherapy as a powerful weapon you have chosen to use to fight the cancer. This may make the side effects a little more bearable. But feeling depressed or anxious is normal, and nothing to be ashamed of. Asking for help is not always easy; talk to someone else on the team if your specialist seems too busy to spare the time.

3

YOU REALLY NEED TO KNOW

◆ The most serious side effect of chemotherapy is weakening of the immune system, which increases the risk of infection.

◆ Other side effects can be rather unpleasant, but are not dangerous.

◆ Most side effects of chemotherapy are not permanent.

Systemic therapy

Systemic therapy

Hormone therapy

The growth of some breast cancers is influenced by hormones, especially estrogen. A test can be done on a sample of the cancer to see if the cells contain what are called hormone receptors (estrogen receptors and progesterone receptors). If the cancer cells do contain one or both types of receptor, it is a "receptor-positive" cancer, and hormone therapy has a high chance of success. In general, receptor-positive cancers have a better outlook than receptor-negative cancers. If the cancer cells are receptor-negative, hormone therapy will not work, and your doctor will recommend chemotherapy.

The most common hormone therapy used in breast cancer is the drug tamoxifen, which blocks estrogen. It works best for postmenopausal women with hormone receptor-positive tumors. For this group, it may be the only adjuvant therapy needed.

Tamoxifen is taken as a tablet, usually 20 milligrams once a day. The recommendations at present are that you take it for five years. In the future, this may be extended, when more is known about its long-term side effects.

Tamoxifen may also benefit premenopausal women, although to a lesser extent than women over 50. This is why it is used following chemotherapy in treating younger women. Although tamoxifen cures fewer breast cancers in women under 50, it lengthens the time before possible recurrence. Younger women get less benefit from tamoxifen because they tend to have hormone receptor-negative breast cancer, and because their ovaries are still producing estrogen.

What are the side effects?

The side effects of tamoxifen are relatively rare and mild. Because of its effect on estrogen, it can cause menopausal symptoms, such as hot flushes, vaginal dryness, vaginal discharge, and weight gain. There is a slightly increased chance of getting a deep vein thrombosis (a blood clot in your calf), and there is also a slightly increased risk of developing cataracts (damage to the lens of the eye that blurs vision).

The most serious effect of tamoxifen is the increased risk of developing endometrial cancer (cancer of the lining of the womb). Women who take hormone replacement therapy (HRT) share this risk, but the risks need to be weighed against the benefits. The chances of a woman with breast cancer developing endometrial cancer after taking tamoxifen are much smaller than the chances of her developing a second breast cancer if she does not take tamoxifen. It is reassuring to know that you can have check-ups for endometrial cancer; these include a yearly examination and regular ultrasound scans of the womb. You should also watch out for irregular or abnormal bleeding or very heavy periods and report them to your doctor as soon as possible.

YOU REALLY NEED TO KNOW

◆ Hormone therapy improves survival rate and can cure some breast cancers.

◆ Tamoxifen increases your risk of endometrial cancer threefold, but greatly reduces the risk of developing a second breast cancer.

Systemic therapy

Systemic therapy

Positive side effects

Tamoxifen also has beneficial side effects, such as protecting against osteoporosis (thinning of the bones) and heart disease. The biggest advantage is that it halves your chances of getting breast cancer in your other breast. Recent studies have also shown that for certain women at high risk for breast cancer, tamoxifen can reduce the risk of breast cancer developing in the first place by 40% in five years.

Removal of the ovaries

Surgery to remove the ovaries (oophorectomy) changes the levels of hormones in the body, which in turn has an effect on how breast cancer behaves. Oophorectomy was first used to treat breast cancer in the 1940s, but was performed less and less as combinations of drugs for chemotherapy were developed and the treatment became

GENETIC RESEARCH AND BREAST CANCER

The HERZ/neu mutation

Research is currently uncovering genetic changes that play a part in the development of breast cancer. For example, about 20 to 30 percent of breast cancers are associated with what is known as the HERZ/neu gene mutation. A certain sequence on a gene, given the name HERZ/neu, stimulates cancer cells to grow. The recently developed drug trastuzumab (Herceptin) helps to block the effects of the HERZ/neu gene product, making use of the body's own immune system.

more popular. These days, oopherectomy in pre-menopausal women with breast cancer significantly improves how long women can survive their cancer.

The disadvantage of oophorectomy is that it causes immediate menopause. Women who are at very high risk of recurrence may choose to give up their ability to have children—or to have more children—to improve their chances of a cure.

Prophylactic mastectomy

In any disease, prevention is better than cure. This is especially true when you are dealing with life-threatening cancer, and there is a lot of research aimed at breast cancer prevention, also called prophylaxis.

Women who are at very high risk of breast cancer may consider having a double mastectomy to try to prevent it from developing. This is a dramatic and irreversible step, and the decision takes time to make, but if you have lost more than one close family member to breast cancer or tests show that you have a gene that carries a high risk of breast cancer (see p. 17), and you are very worried about developing the disease yourself, having prophylactic mastectomies may give you some peace of mind. Also, if you are at high risk and your breasts are not easy to examine or your mammograms are not easy to interpret—perhaps because your breasts are very large or small—you may want to consider having the operation.

The decision to have this drastic surgery should never be made in a hurry. Take six months to go through all your options, get counseling, and discuss the pros and cons fully with your partner, family, and friends before finally deciding to go ahead.

Systemic therapy

Chapter

4

LIVING WITH CANCER

Looking and feeling good

✔ After a radical mastectomy the arm on the affected side will be permanently weakened because the muscles of the chest wall have been removed, but exercise will improve mobility.

✔ Try to exercise for short periods every day rather than longer, less frequent sessions.

EVERYDAY EXERCISES

After surgery you will need to exercise your arm and shoulder to get full movement back. Exercises will usually be recommended by the physical therapist in the hospital as early as the second day after surgery. Follow medical advice and do not try to do too much too soon. The exercises illustrated below can safely be done at home.

◆ Rotate your shoulder on the affected side in a circular motion, leaving your arm hanging by your side.

◆ Rest your elbow on the affected side on a firm surface and brush your hair.

◆ Hold a tennis ball in your hand on the affected side (above) and squeeze and release it a few times, increasing the number of times as your strength returns.

◆ Practice strapping your bra, clasping your hands behind your back and then stretching them out sideways.

◆ Hold a large towel with one hand over your shoulder and the other behind your waist. Dry your back using a series of long, slow, diagonal movements, then change hands.

◆ Hold a beanbag in one hand, lift it, and drop it behind your back (left), catching it with your other hand. Repeat with the other arm. You can make a beanbag out of a sock.

◆ Hold each end of a rope hanging over a door. Sit with the door between your knees. Pull the rope with one hand so the other arm goes up, then pull that arm down, and so on.

◆ Lean on the back of a chair, with your forehead resting on your good arm (left). Let your weak arm hang loosely, then swing it back and forth, side to side, and around and around.

YOU REALLY NEED TO KNOW

◆ It is important to exercise your arm and shoulder after surgery so that you regain full movement.

◆ Always follow medical advice and do not try to do too much too soon.

Looking and feeling good

Breast prosthesis

Worrying about your appearance and wanting to look as good as you can are normal feelings. Some women think they are being vain if they ask about prostheses or wigs during treatment for cancer. But self-image and emotional well-being are important, and if wearing a wig or an attractive outfit makes you feel better, it is worth it, especially since there is evidence that your state of mind plays an important role in the outcome of your treatment.

A breast prosthesis is a false breast, which may or may not have a nipple. If you have decided against reconstruction, or are still in the process of making up your mind, you may want to find out about prostheses.

CHOOSING THE PROSTHESIS FOR YOU

There are many different shapes, colors, and sizes of prosthesis available, as well as a variety of nipples. Breast forms can also be custom made. Your health insurance booklet will outline what is covered in your case.

All women who have had a mastectomy are strongly recommended to try out a properly fitted, weighted breast form. Before leaving the hospital, you should have been given the opportunity to wear a much lighter, temporary prosthesis, while your scar was healing.

Within four to six weeks of surgery you will be ready to be fitted for a permanent prosthesis. Prostheses are made from silicone, and have the same weight and feel as a natural breast. They last for two to four years. Silicone is waterproof and can be worn safely during most activities.

Some prostheses can be attached directly to the skin with an adhesive strip. Others slip into a pocket in a special bra, which may be soft-cup or underwire. The bras are made with wider straps and a larger underband than regular bras, and are available in several different styles and colors.

You will be able to wear most styles of clothing. Special bathing suits are available, although you may still be able to wear an ordinary one. Someone on your medical team should be able to give you information about where you can go for all the supplies you need.

Wigs

If your treatment includes chemotherapy, you may lose some or all of your hair. It is a good idea to think about what you would like to do before this happens. Some women find it boosts their morale to have an attractive wig ready before chemotherapy starts—perhaps even to radically change their hair color or style. Your breast care nurse or someone else on your team will be able to advise you on where to get one. Alternatively, you might like to experiment with different hats and scarves.

YOU REALLY NEED TO KNOW

◆ Self-image and emotional well-being are important, so do not be afraid to ask for information about prostheses and wigs.

◆ Prostheses are available in different materials and skin tones, and in a wide selection of shapes and sizes. They can also be custom made.

Looking and feeling good

After treatment

Once treatment is over you may be surprised to feel rather lost—the period of activity and doing something about your illness is gone and you no longer have regular contact with all the familiar medical staff. You may feel unsupported, at the very time when you are adjusting to the physical and psychological changes that have taken place. It's normal to feel sad for the loss of the person you were before your illness. Take all the time you need to come to terms with the fact that the changes are permanent. Many women find it helps to have an outlet for their feelings. This could be your regular doctor, a psychologist, a religious counselor, or a support group.

Your sexual self

For many people, sex is a very important part of their relationship, yet it is one that is rarely talked about openly and candidly. But when a serious illness affects one

Many women worry that their partner will find them less attractive after breast surgery, but a lot of couples find that the experience of tackling breast cancer together strengthens the bond between them.

partner, it is vital to talk about the affect it will have on a couple's sex life. Having sex again after a major life change such as treatment for breast cancer is never easy and may be awkward and embarrassing at first. If you have had a mastectomy or chemotherapy you may feel sensitive about your changed appearance.

Set a time to talk to your partner and to listen to what he has to say. You may not feel ready for intercourse, but try to be specific about what you are prepared and want to do. Often a cuddle and a hug will be enough to bring you closer. Gradually you will feel ready to move on to a wider range of sexual activities.

Accepting the new you

In time, you will come to accept your new shape, and feel proud of what you have achieved. Your choices about reconstruction, prosthesis, and clothing are all part of the process of reaffirming yourself as a woman. Each individual experience is unique, but the strength and support gained from sharing your concerns with others in the same position, or with a counselor, can speed up the recovery and healing processes.

What about recurrence?

When surgery and any adjuvant treatment are completed, your cancer may be in remission. You will be relieved, but now comes a different type of stress.

You and your doctor need to be on the lookout for recurrence, especially during the next five years. You need to make a clear plan for follow-up and review, with regular appointments for the first two years, and then twice yearly, including an annual mammogram and a chest X-ray.

YOU REALLY NEED TO KNOW

◆ Life after treatment will certainly be different, but it can be both positive and rewarding.

◆ You can have a happy and fulfilling sex life after breast cancer treatment.

◆ You need to have regular check-ups for the first two years and then yearly mammograms and chest X-rays.

After treatment

After treatment

✓ Research shows that your state of mind may play a role in boosting your body's natural defenses against cancer.

✗ Some alternative therapies are known to be beneficial, but others may have a damaging effect on the outcome of conventional treatment or may even be dangerous.

What about support?

You should know who to phone if you are concerned about anything. Having this structure in place can be reassuring, but many women experience periods of extreme anxiety and fear that their cancer has returned. If these feelings become overwhelming, you may need help from your doctor. Anxiety and depression can be treated with counseling and antidepressant drugs, so do say so if you are feeling down or are unusually tearful or irritable, if your appetite has changed, or if you are having difficulty sleeping.

Living your life

Treatment for breast cancer can be uncomfortable and exhausting. Looking forward and making plans to enjoy life once your treatment is over will help to make the

In the future, all breast cancer centers may offer a range of complementary and alternative therapies alongside the traditional treatments. Until then you can find out what is available in your area from your doctor's office or a breast cancer support group.

discomfort easier to bear. It is important to look after yourself and to get involved in activities that you find rewarding. Many women find that their attitude to life has changed—for example, little problems may no longer seem so important. You might decide to do something you have always wanted to do but never got around to or you may simply want to get back to your normal routine—family, friends, and work commitments—as quickly as possible. Whatever your choices, give yourself time to adjust to this new phase of life. Breast cancer is a major crisis in any woman's life, and physical and emotional recovery take time.

Complementary therapies

Therapies that "complement" conventional medicine and can be used with it, such as homeopathy, massage, and aromatherapy, are known as complementary. Alternative therapies, such as herbalism, are not usually used alongside conventional medicine. You may be interested in finding out whether any of these therapies suit you. But remember when exploring the options that it is important—even if you are feeling disappointed or fed up with your current treatment program—to let your specialist or the breast care nurse know which other therapies you want to try.

The modern approach to cancer treatment is for doctors to encourage any complementary therapies that have a positive impact on the patient. Therapies being used include visualization techniques, meditation and relaxation, acupuncture, and vitamin supplements. However, no responsible complementary or alternative practitioner should ever advise you to stop all other treatments or claim to offer a "cure" for cancer.

YOU REALLY NEED TO KNOW

◆ Talking about your experiences and worries will help you come to terms with them.

◆ There are breast cancer counselors and support groups that can give you help and support when you need it.

◆ Not all alternative therapies are harmless, so get as much information and advice as possible before you try any different type of treatment.

After treatment

Talking to children

✓ Children often accept body changes more easily than adults do.

✓ Some children may try to be extra good; others may behave badly as they try to cope with the news.

✓ Some children may feel sorry for themselves, then feel guilty because they think they should feel sorry for you.

You may feel you want to protect your children by not telling them about your breast cancer for as long as possible, but you should avoid this temptation. Even young children know when something is wrong, and if they are not told the truth, they can feel isolated and more anxious. Children also have an amazing capacity for dealing with unpleasant facts.

When should I tell my children?

Talk to your children as soon as you have been diagnosed with breast cancer. The amount of detail you go into will depend on their ages and how easy you find it to talk about your cancer. Explain what is wrong and what your treatment will involve, including any possible side effects. You may find it easier to talk to your children individually at this stage.

Talk about your treatment

Keep your children informed as your treatment progresses, without going into too much detail. If you are going to have chemotherapy, for example, warn your children that your hair will fall out and tell them that it will grow back in time. Tell them also that you will be very tired while your treatment is happening, but try to spend time with them doing activities that are not too tiring, such as watching TV or playing board games.

Children's worries

You will need to be sensitive to your children's reactions. Younger children may worry that they have caused your cancer or that they might catch it. Reassure them that cancer is an illness that is not caused by anyone, nor is it contagious. Remember, information is power.

PLAN WHAT YOU WILL SAY

Before you tell your children about your cancer, it may help to plan what you are going to say and how you will say it.

DO...

◆ Avoid medical terms—use language your children can easily understand.

◆ Listen to your children to find out how much information they can cope with at any one time.

◆ Be truthful—children know when you are hiding something from them.

◆ Correct any mistaken ideas they may have.

◆ Try to keep your home routine as normal as possible.

◆ Let your children's school know what is happening.

◆ Tell your children honestly how you feel.

◆ Remember it's okay to cry—for you and your children.

◆ Be prepared to repeat information and to answer questions as often as your children need.

◆ Stress the positive whenever you can.

◆ Use dolls and role play to explain the situation to a younger child.

◆ Contact a support group and get together with other families who are coping with cancer (see p. 78).

DON'T...

◆ Be afraid to say "I don't know."

◆ Hide your emotions—honesty is the best policy.

◆ Give children too many medical details.

◆ Push your children to talk if they are not ready.

◆ Make promises unless you are sure you can keep them.

YOU REALLY NEED TO KNOW

◆ Children have the right to know about things that affect the family—such as a new diagnosis of cancer.

◆ Teenagers may find it particularly hard to cope with their emotions when they are told.

◆ Some children may be afraid that they, too, will develop cancer.

◆ If you don't tell your children the truth, they may learn it from someone else, or get misleading information from other sources.

Talking to children

Palliative care

DID YOU KNOW?

✓ People who need strong pain medication do get used to having high doses; this is to be expected and is perfectly acceptable.

✓ Palliative care is about fulfilling the physical, emotional, spiritual, and financial needs of those who know they are dying.

In some cases, the breast cancer may recur and progress despite treatment. If that happens and a cure is no longer possible, the objective of all treatment and support becomes the control of any symptoms you may develop. This is called palliative care, a branch of medicine that focuses on the quality of life for patients who cannot be cured. Palliative care aims to strike the right balance between trying to extend life at all costs and trying to make the end of a terminal illness as peaceful as possible.

Accepting the inevitable

Death and dying are not subjects that most of us feel comfortable talking or thinking about. Knowing that you have a life-threatening disease means you have probably thought more about it than others, but you may still find it difficult to talk about, especially to your loved ones. There comes a time for some women with breast cancer when everybody, from the patient to her family and the team looking after her, will need to adjust to the knowledge that the disease is now terminal.

Possible reactions

You may go through a number of different reactions. You may experience shock or disbelief; you may become very angry; you may be very frightened; some people even feel guilty (although nobody should); and some people just cannot take in the reality.

Coming to terms with your illness will take time. You may feel lonely and afraid along the way, and find that your priorities change with time, but it can help to share your fears with other breast cancer sufferers, a counselor, and your family and friends. Having some

WHAT A HOSPICE CAN OFFER

Hospices can help with many aspects of your disease, from pain management to tips on preparing food and skin care after surgery. They also provide support and counseling, both to the patient and her family. You may want financial or legal advice to help you get your affairs in order, or to discuss your religious and spiritual needs. The hospice can help with all of these, more so than a hospital, because the staff have time and training to focus on the specific needs of cancer patients.

The old-fashioned view of hospices as places people go to die is fading, but you may still feel shocked if your doctor suggests you contact a hospice. The modern role of hospices includes caring for cancer patients at home as well as providing in-patient care.

idea of how to handle the inevitable end and making plans helps both patients and their family and friends cope better. When everything is settled and everyone knows what you want, you may not need to talk about the subject ever again.

Controlling pain

Nowadays, really effective pain control can be achieved for the vast majority of patients. The most important message to remember is that most pain, whether mild or severe, short-term or long-term, can be well controlled and there is no need to suffer. If your doctor does not know what services are available locally, contact one of the organizations listed on p. 78 for advice.

Palliative care

Understanding the jargon

Many of the terms that you will meet when finding out more about breast cancer may be unfamiliar to you. This page gives definitions of the words you are most likely to come across.

ADJUVANT—treatment used in addition to surgery.

AXILLA—the armpit.

BENIGN—a tumor that grows in one place and does not spread to any other part of the body.

BIOPSY—the removal of a piece of tissue from the body for examination under a microscope.

CHEMOTHERAPY—the use of drugs to destroy cancer cells throughout the body.

CYTOLOGY—the examination of cells under the microscope to look for evidence of disease.

DYSPLASIA—abnormal cell growth.

GENE—a piece of DNA that contains information that controls how cells behave.

HORMONE—a chemical in the body that influences how cells and body systems work.

HYPERPLASIA—overgrowth of cells.

IN SITU—tumor growth that has not invaded any of the surrounding tissue.

LUMPECTOMY—surgical removal of a breast lump.

LYMPH NODE—part of the lymphatic system that becomes enlarged when affected by disease.

LYMPHEDEMA—swelling (for example of the arm) when lymph drainage becomes blocked, especially after radiotherapy.

MALIGNANT—cancer that invades the surrounding tissue and other areas of the body.

MAMMOGRAM—X-ray of the breast.

MASTECTOMY—surgical removal of the breast.

METASTASIS—spread of cancer from the primary site to a secondary site in the body.

OOPHORECTOMY—surgical removal of the ovaries.

PALLIATIVE TREATMENT—treating the symptoms of terminal disease in order to improve quality of life.

PRIMARY CANCER—the original tumor before any spread took place.

REMISSION—when a disease is present but not active, for example after treatment.

SECONDARIES—tumors that grow as a result of spreading (also called metastases).

SYSTEMIC—treatment that reaches all the systems of the body, not just the breast.

TUMOR—an abnormal growth or lump, which may be benign or malignant.

Understanding the jargon

Useful addresses

ROSE KUSHNER BREAST CANCER ADVISORY CENTER
P.O. Box 224
Kensington, MD 20895
Tel: (301) 897-3445
Fax: (301) 897-3444
Founded in 1975; information service for people concerned with breast cancer. Publishes If You've Ever Thought about Breast Cancer *by Rose Kushner, biennial. Free.*

SUSAN G. KOMEN BREAST CANCER FOUNDATION
5005 LBJ, Suite 370
Dallas, TX 75244
Tel: (972) 385-5005
1-800-IM-AWARE
Fax: (972) 385-5005
www.breastcancerinfo.com
Founded in 1982; 1,000 members. Free quarterly newsletter, Frontline, *highlights current breast cancer issues and Komen events. Comprehensive organization: advocacy, public awareness, funding through grants for research, and screening programs. Sponsors educational programs, speakers' bureau, awards, research center.*

Y-ME NATIONAL BREAST CANCER CENTER
c/o Sharon Green
212 W. Van Buren
Chicago, IL 60607
Tel: (312) 986-8338
HOTLINE: 1-800-221-2141
Fax: (312) 294-8597
email: YMEONE@aol.com
www.y-me.org
Founded in 1978; 4,600 members. Provides peer support and information to women who have or suspect they have breast cancer. Activities—presurgical counseling and referral service, programs for professionals including hotline volunteer training. Bimonthly newsletter, Y-ME Hotline, *and publications including* For Single Women with Breast Cancer *and* When the Woman You Love Has Breast Cancer.

REACH TO RECOVER
c/o American Cancer Society
1599 Clifton Road NE
Atlanta, GA 30329
1-800-ACS-2345
Fax (404) 636-5567
www.cancer.org
A one-on-one visitation program for information and support for women with breast cancer concerns. The Reach to Recover counselor gives information and practical, not medical, advice.

Index

Index

Acknowledgments

Photographs: Amoena (UK) ltd 66; Marshall Editions/Iain Bagwell 26/27; Science Photo Library (Breast Screening Unit, Kings College Hospital, London) 31, (Colin Cuthbert) 57, (Cecil H. Fox) 36/37, 45, 51, 73, (Simon Fraser) 46, (Dr. P. Marazzi) 41, (Larry Mulvehill) 52; N1H Custom Medical Stock Photo 34, 75, (Chris Priest) 24/25; (Quest) 7, 22, 39, 48, (Geoff Tompkinson) 28; gettyone Stone 17

Commissioned photography: Guglielmo Galvin

Edited and designed by Phoebus Editions, 72–80 Leather Lane, London EC1N 7TR

Thanks to Patsy North and Ros Newby for modelling for the photographs.